Coconut

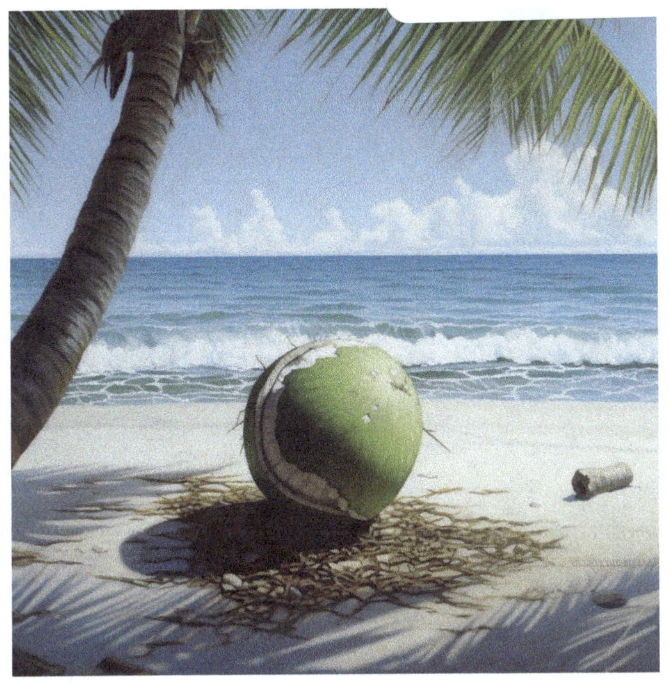

H.-G. Saenger

The Book:

"Coconut: A Journey through the History, Cultivation and Uses of the Tropical Stone Fruit" takes you on an insightful journey into the fascinating world of the coconut. The book aims to provide a comprehensive understanding of this unique fruit, covering its origin, history, cultivation, uses and cultural significance. It also explores the coconut's potential for sustainable development and its role in the modern world.

The Author:

H.-G. Saenger
Passionate reader
and versatile author.
Lives since 2020 with his second wife
wife in Thailand

Coconut

The remarkable world of the coconut

by

H.-G. Saenger

- 1 -

1. Edition, 2023

© 2023 All rights reserved.

No.4/2 Moo.7

A.Mueang Ban Khok

67000 Phetchabun

H.-G. Saenger

Table of Contents:

Introduction: The Remarkable World of Coconuts

Throughout history, coconuts have served as a vital source of sustenance, economic wealth, and cultural identity for millions of people across the tropical regions of the world. The coconut palm (Cocos nucifera) is often referred to as the „Tree of Life" due to the multitude of uses derived from its various parts, including the fruit, leaves, husk, and trunk. This incredible versatility has led to its widespread cultivation and use across a diverse range of cultures and geographies.

„**Coconuts:** A Journey through the History, Cultivation, and Uses of the Tropical Drupes" takes you on an enlightening voyage into the fascinating world of coconuts. The book aims to provide a comprehensive understanding of this unique fruit, covering its origins, history, cultivation, uses, and cultural significance. It also explores the coconut's potential for sustainable development and its role in the modern world.

In the first few chapters, the book delves into the origins and early history of coconuts, tracing their journey from their ancestral home in the Indo-Pacific region to their eventual spread across the globe. It highlights the extraordinary ability of coconuts to adapt to diverse environments and the vital role they played in the development of ancient maritime trade routes.

The book also delves into the anatomy of the coconut palm, shedding light on its unique characteristics and the factors that contribute to its unparalleled versatility. From there, the focus shifts to the cultivation and farming techniques employed by coconut farmers, as well as the harvesting and processing methods used to extract the fruit's various components.

As the book progresses, it examines the many uses of coconuts, from their culinary and medicinal applications to their industrial and personal care applications. The discussion includes the health benefits associated with coconut consumption, such as their potential to lower cholesterol, aid digestion, and boost the immune system.

In addition to examining the various uses of coconuts, the book also addresses the environmental impact and sustainability of coconut production. It evaluates the challenges faced by the coconut industry, including deforestation, loss of biodiversity, and the exploitation of small-scale farmers. The book also presents potential solutions to these issues, such as the adoption of sustainable farming practices, fair trade initiatives, and support for small-scale producers.

The role of coconuts in culture and folklore is another fascinating aspect explored in this book. From their symbolism in religious ceremonies to their portrayal in popular media, coconuts have captured the imagination of countless generations. The book also offers a glimpse into the future of coconuts, highlighting new discoveries and innovations in coconut-based products and technologies.

Finally, the book concludes with a collection of delicious coconut recipes, providing readers with a chance to experience the diverse flavors and textures of this remarkable fruit. By the end of this journey, you will have gained a newfound appreciation for the humble coconut and its incredible potential to nourish, heal, and sustain communities around the world.

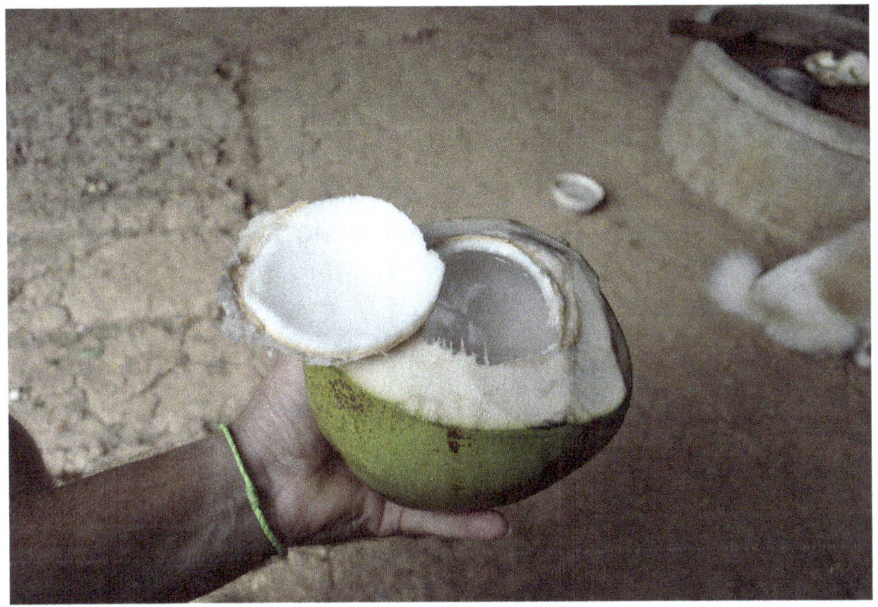

Chapter 1: The Origins and Early History of Coconuts

The story of coconuts begins in the vast expanse of the Indo-Pacific region, where the coconut palm (Cocos nucifera) is believed to have first evolved. Though the exact origin of the coconut palm is still debated among scientists, it is generally accepted that the species originated either in the Indian Ocean's islands or the western Pacific's coastal areas. Genetic studies have helped narrow down these potential origins, but the mystery remains unsolved.

The coconut's remarkable ability to float on water played a crucial role in its dispersal across the globe. The fruit's hard, buoyant husk allowed it to drift thousands of miles across oceans, eventually reaching the shores of distant lands. Over time, the coconut palm became a familiar sight on the coastlines of Asia, Africa, and the Americas, adapting to diverse environments and thriving in the tropical climates of these regions.

The early history of coconuts is intertwined with the development of ancient maritime trade routes. Evidence suggests that coconuts were utilized by seafaring cultures such as the Austronesians and Indo-Aryans, who began to trade and cultivate the fruit more than 2,000 years ago. These maritime traders played a pivotal role in the spread of coconuts throughout the Indian Ocean, Southeast Asia, and the Pacific Islands.

One of the earliest known references to coconuts can be found in the Indian epic, the Ramayana, which dates back to the 5th century BCE. The fruit is also mentioned in ancient Sanskrit texts, signifying its cultural importance in early Indian societies. Similarly, ancient Polynesians are believed to have relied on coconuts as a vital source of sustenance during their long ocean voyages, using the fruit's various parts for food, drink, and shelter.

As coconuts became more widely cultivated and traded, their uses expanded beyond mere sustenance. In India, for example, coconuts were used in religious ceremonies and as a symbol of prosperity, while in the Philippines, the leaves of the coconut palm were woven into textiles and used for roofing materials. This resourcefulness exemplifies the ingenuity of early human societies and their ability to harness the full potential of this versatile fruit.

The early history of coconuts also played a role in the establishment of colonial empires. European explorers like Marco Polo, who encountered the coconut during his travels in the 13th century, brought back stories of the exotic fruit, which sparked curiosity and interest among European societies. Later, European colonizers recognized the economic potential of coconuts and sought to exploit their cultivation and trade.

By the 19th century, coconuts had become an essential crop in many colonial territories, with large-scale plantations established throughout Southeast Asia, Africa, and the Caribbean. This period marked a significant turning point in the history of coconuts, as their cultivation shifted from small-scale, local production to a globalized industry driven by profit and colonial interests.

In summary, the origins and early history of coconuts demonstrate the fruit's remarkable journey from its ancestral home in the Indo-Pacific region to its widespread cultivation and use across the globe. The coconut's unique characteristics, coupled with human ingenuity, have led to its enduring presence in the tropical regions of the world and its lasting cultural, economic, and culinary significance.

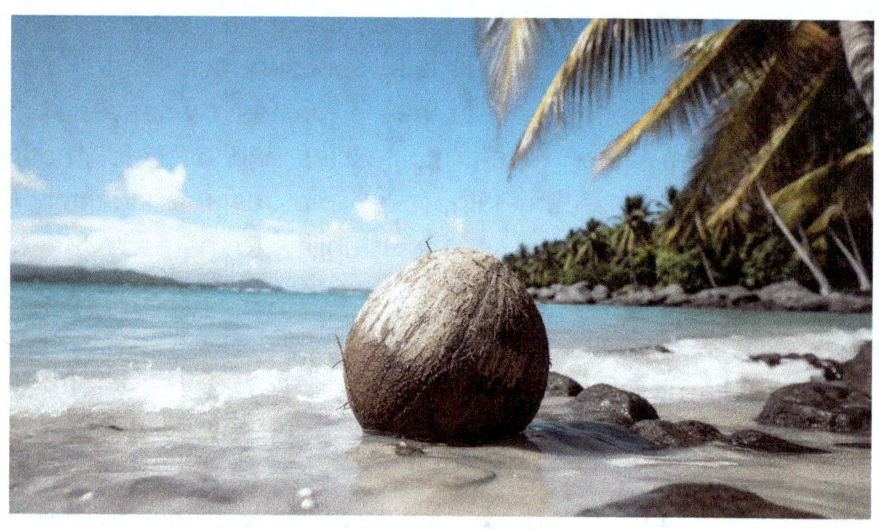

Chapter 2: The Spread of Coconuts Around the Globe

The dispersal of coconuts around the world is an intriguing tale of natural processes and human intervention, which has led to the widespread cultivation and use of this versatile fruit across diverse cultures and geographies.

Natural Dispersal:

As mentioned in the previous chapter, one of the most significant factors that contributed to the spread of coconuts was their unique ability to float on water. The coconut's hard, buoyant husk enabled the fruit to drift for thousands of miles across the ocean, surviving long periods without losing its viability. This natural dispersal mechanism allowed coconuts to colonize the coastlines of the Indian Ocean, Southeast Asia, the Pacific Islands, and eventually the shores of Africa and the Americas.

In some instances, this process of natural dispersal was facilitated by ocean currents and prevailing winds. For example, the eastward-flowing Equatorial Counter Current played a crucial role in transporting coconuts from the Indo-Pacific region to the tropical coastlines of Central and South America. Similarly, the westward-flowing South Equatorial Current carried coconuts across the Indian Ocean, enabling the fruit to establish itself on the eastern coast of Africa.

Human Intervention:

While natural dispersal played a significant role in the spread of coconuts, human intervention also contributed to the fruit's global distribution. Ancient maritime traders and explorers, such as the Austronesians and Indo-Aryans, were instrumental in the dissemination of coconuts throughout the Indian Ocean, Southeast Asia, and the Pacific Islands.

These seafaring cultures recognized the value of coconuts as a source of sustenance and materials, and began cultivating the fruit in their settlements. As their trade networks expanded, so too did the cultivation of coconuts, which were often planted along trade routes and coastal settlements to ensure a steady supply for travelers and traders.

European Exploration and Colonization:

The arrival of European explorers in the 15th century marked a new phase in the spread of coconuts. Upon encountering the fruit during their travels, explorers like Marco Polo and Vasco da Gama brought back tales of the exotic coconut, sparking curiosity and interest among European societies.

Subsequently, European colonizers recognized the economic potential of coconuts and sought to exploit their cultivation and trade. As a result, large-scale coconut plantations were established throughout Southeast Asia, Africa, and the Caribbean during the colonial era. This period saw a significant shift in coconut cultivation, transforming it from small-scale, local production to a globalized industry driven by profit and colonial interests.

Modern Distribution:

Today, coconuts are cultivated in more than 90 countries across the tropical belt, with the largest producers being Indonesia, the Philippines, and India. The global spread of coconuts has led to the development of numerous varieties and cultivars, each with its unique characteristics, suited to the specific environmental conditions of their respective regions.

In conclusion, the spread of coconuts around the globe is a testament to the fruit's remarkable adaptability and its enduring appeal to diverse cultures and societies. Through a combination of natural dispersal, human intervention, and historical factors, coconuts have become an integral part of the tropical landscape and a vital source of sustenance and wealth for millions of people worldwide.

Chapter 3: The Anatomy of the Coconut Palm

The coconut palm (Cocos nucifera) is a remarkable plant, not only for its fruit but also for the various uses derived from its different parts. To better understand the versatility of the coconut palm, it is essential to examine its anatomy and the unique characteristics that contribute to its wide range of applications.

Trunk: The coconut palm's trunk is tall, slender, and slightly curved, typically reaching heights of 20-30 meters (66-98 feet). The trunk is covered in distinctive rings, which are the scars left behind by fallen leaves. The trunk is sturdy and flexible, making it a suitable material for construction, particularly in regions where timber is scarce. It is commonly used for building houses, bridges, and furniture, among other things.

Leaves: The coconut palm's large, feather-like leaves, called fronds, can grow up to 6 meters (20 feet) in length. The fronds are pinnately compound, consisting of numerous leaflets arranged along a central axis. The leaves serve a variety of purposes, including thatching for roofs, making baskets, and weaving mats. The leaf midribs, known as ribs, can also be used as brooms or for constructing fences.

Inflorescence: The coconut palm's inflorescence is a branching, flower-bearing structure known as a spadix. Each spadix consists of multiple spikelets, which contain both male and female flowers. The male flowers are more numerous and produce pollen, while the female flowers, situated at the base of the spikelets, develop into coconuts. In some traditional cultures, the sap collected from the inflorescence is used to produce a sweet, nutritious beverage called „tuba" or „toddy," which can be fermented to create alcoholic drinks or further processed into vinegar or sugar.

Fruit: The coconut fruit, also known as a drupe, is the most widely utilized part of the coconut palm. The fruit consists of several layers:

a. Exocarp: The outermost layer, or exocarp, is smooth and green when the fruit is immature, turning brown as it ripens.

b. Mesocarp: The middle layer, or mesocarp, is composed of fibrous husk material called coir. Coir is used to produce a variety of products, including ropes, mats, and brushes, as well as for horticultural purposes as a soil amendment or growing medium.

c. Endocarp: The innermost layer, or endocarp, is the hard, woody shell that encloses the coconut's edible part. The shell can be used to create handicrafts, utensils, and decorative items.

d. Endosperm: The endosperm is the edible part of the coconut, which consists of two components: the white, fleshy „meat" called copra, and the clear liquid known as coconut water. Copra is rich in healthy fats and is used for producing coconut oil, milk, and flour, while coconut water is a refreshing and hydrating beverage.

Roots: The coconut palm has a fibrous root system, which helps anchor the tree in sandy soils and allows it to absorb water and nutrients efficiently. In some traditional societies, the roots are used for medicinal purposes or as a natural dye.

In conclusion, the anatomy of the coconut palm reveals the plant's remarkable versatility and resourcefulness. Each part of the palm serves a distinct purpose, contributing to the coconut palm's status as the „Tree of Life" and providing a multitude of uses for the people who cultivate and rely upon it.

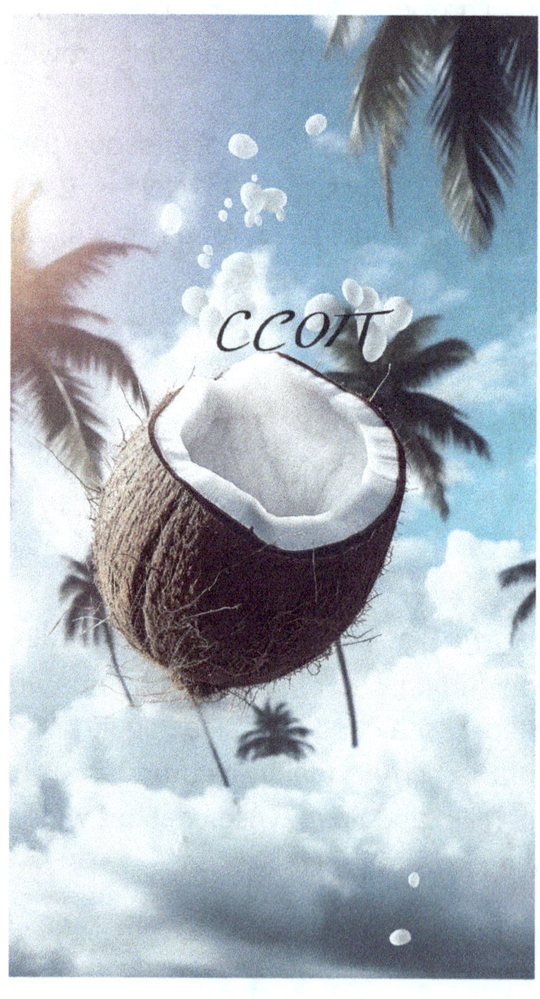

Chapter 4: Coconut Cultivation and Farming Techniques

Coconut cultivation is an essential source of livelihood for millions of people in tropical regions around the world. The process of cultivating coconut palms and harvesting their fruit requires specialized knowledge, skills, and techniques to ensure the health, productivity, and sustainability of the trees. This chapter explores the various aspects of coconut cultivation, from planting and caring for the trees to harvesting and processing the fruit.

Site selection: The coconut palm thrives in well-drained, sandy or loamy soils with a pH of 5.5 to 7.0. Ideally, the plantation site should be near the coastline, as coconut palms are salt-tolerant and can benefit from the sea breeze. Additionally, the site should receive plenty of sunlight and have a warm, humid climate with ample rainfall.

Planting: Coconut palms can be propagated from seedlings, which are typically obtained from healthy, high-yielding mother trees. The seedlings are usually around 9-12 months old when they are ready for transplanting. Planting holes should be at least 60 cm (24 inches) deep and wide, with a spacing of 7.5-9 meters (25-30 feet) between trees to allow for adequate growth and sunlight penetration. The seedlings should be planted with the pointed end of the nut facing downwards, ensuring that the top one-third of the nut is above the soil surface.

Irrigation and drainage: Coconut palms require regular irrigation, particularly during the early stages of growth and during dry periods. Drip irrigation systems are commonly used to provide consistent moisture without causing waterlogging, which can be detrimental to the trees. Proper drainage is also crucial to prevent root rot and other diseases associated with excess moisture.

Fertilization: Coconut palms benefit from the application of both organic and inorganic fertilizers. Organic matter, such as compost or manure, helps improve soil structure and nutrient availability. Inorganic fertilizers, particularly those containing nitrogen, phosphorus, and potassium, can be applied to enhance tree growth and fruit production. It is essential to follow recommended application rates and timings to prevent nutrient imbalances and potential harm to the environment.

Pest and disease management: Coconut palms are susceptible to various pests and diseases, which can negatively impact their growth and yield. Integrated pest management (IPM) strategies, including the use of biological controls, cultural practices, and chemical treatments, can help minimize the impact of these threats. Regular monitoring and early detection of pests and diseases are crucial to prevent significant damage and ensure the health of the trees.

Pruning and maintenance: Periodic pruning of coconut palms can improve their productivity and overall health. Removing dead or damaged fronds, as well as excess fruit bunches, can promote better light penetration and air circulation within the canopy. This practice also helps reduce the risk of pest and disease infestations.

Harvesting: Coconuts are generally harvested at different stages of maturity, depending on their intended use. Green coconuts, which contain a high volume of refreshing coconut water, are harvested around six to seven months after pollination. Mature coconuts, characterized by their brown husks and firm, white flesh, are harvested around 11-12 months after pollination. Harvesting methods vary, with some farmers using long poles, climbing the trees, or employing trained monkeys to collect the fruit.

Post-harvest processing: After harvesting, coconuts undergo various processing steps, depending on their intended use. For example, the husks can be removed to extract the fibrous coir, which is used to make ropes, mats, and other products. The hard shell is cracked open to obtain the endosperm, which can be processed into copra, coconut milk, or oil. The water inside the coconut can be consumed as a refreshing beverage or used as an ingredient in food and cosmetic products. Proper post-harvest handling and storage are crucial to maintain the quality and safety of coconut products.

Sustainable farming practices: To ensure the long-term viability and environmental sustainability of coconut cultivation, farmers are increasingly adopting sustainable farming practices. These practices include crop diversification, intercropping, and agroforestry, which can enhance soil fertility, reduce pest and disease pressure, and provide additional income sources for farmers. Additionally, conservation of water resources, responsible use of fertilizers and pesticides, and the protection of biodiversity are critical components of sustainable coconut farming.

Climate change and coconut cultivation: Climate change poses significant challenges to coconut cultivation, particularly in terms of changing precipitation patterns, rising temperatures, and increasing frequency of extreme weather events. Adapting to these changes requires innovative solutions, such as the development of climate-resilient coconut varieties, improved water management practices, and the implementation of climate-smart agricultural techniques.

In conclusion, coconut cultivation is a complex and multifaceted process that requires a deep understanding of the coconut palm's biology, environmental requirements, and the diverse techniques used to optimize its growth and productivity. By adopting sustainable farming practices and adapting to the challenges posed by climate change, coconut farmers can help ensure the long-term success and viability of this important crop, which plays a vital role in the economies and cultures of tropical regions worldwide.

Chapter 5: Harvesting and Processing Coconuts

The harvesting and processing of coconuts are essential steps in converting the versatile fruit into a wide array of products that are used for food, health, and industrial applications. This chapter delves into the methods and techniques employed in coconut harvesting and processing, which are crucial for obtaining high-quality products and maximizing their value.

Harvesting Coconuts:

a. Timing: Coconuts can be harvested at various stages of maturity, depending on their intended use. Green coconuts, harvested at around six to seven months after pollination, are valued for their refreshing coconut water. Mature coconuts, harvested at about 11-12 months after pollination, are prized for their firm, white flesh.

b. Methods: Several methods are used for harvesting coconuts, depending on the height of the trees, local traditions, and available resources. Some common methods include:

I. Climbing: Skilled harvesters climb the tree using their hands and feet or a simple harness to reach the fruit. This method is labor-intensive but allows for precise selection of the coconuts to be harvested.

II. Long poles: Harvesters use long poles with a hooked blade or a small net at the end to cut or pull down the coconuts from the ground. This method is less labor-intensive than climbing but may result in damage to the fruit if not executed carefully.

III. Trained animals: In some regions, trained monkeys or even dogs are used to climb the trees and retrieve the coconuts. While this method can be efficient, it raises ethical concerns regarding the treatment of the animals.

Post-harvest Handling:

Proper handling of harvested coconuts is essential to maintain their quality and minimize damage or spoilage. Coconuts should be transported carefully to the processing area, avoiding excessive stacking or pressure that may cause bruising or cracking of the shells. In some cases, the coconuts may be partially processed in the field to reduce transport weight and facilitate further processing.

Processing Coconuts:

The processing of coconuts involves several steps, which vary depending on the intended final product. Some common processing techniques include:

a. Husking: The fibrous outer husk, or mesocarp, is removed using a sharp tool or mechanical dehusker. The extracted coir can be used to produce ropes, mats, brushes, and other products.

b. Shell removal: The hard, woody shell, or endocarp, is cracked open using a specialized tool, such as a machete or a coconut scraper. The separated shells can be used for various purposes, including handicrafts, charcoal production, and as a fuel source.

c. Copra production: The white, fleshy endosperm, or copra, is separated from the shell and typically sun-dried or kiln-dried to reduce its moisture content. Dried copra is then used to produce coconut oil and meal, which is used as animal feed.

d. Coconut milk and cream extraction: Fresh or rehydrated copra is grated and mixed with water, then pressed or squeezed to extract the coconut milk. The milk can be further processed by separating the cream or concentrating it to produce various culinary and cosmetic products.

e. Coconut water: The clear liquid found inside the coconut, known as coconut water, can be consumed as a refreshing beverage or used in the production of various food and cosmetic products. Coconut water is typically collected during the processing of green coconuts.

f. Coconut flour: The residual coconut meal obtained after oil extraction can be further processed to produce coconut flour, a gluten-free alternative to wheat flour used in baking and cooking.

g. Activated charcoal: The shells of coconuts can be processed into activated charcoal, a fine, black, odorless powder with a wide range of applications, including water filtration, air purification, and as a detoxifying agent in health and beauty products.

h. Virgin coconut oil: Virgin coconut oil is extracted from fresh coconut meat without the use of high temperatures or chemicals. This process retains more of the oil's natural nutrients and results in a higher quality product. Virgin coconut oil can be produced using various methods, such as cold pressing, centrifugation, or fermentation.

I. Coconut sugar: The sap collected from the inflorescence of the coconut palm can be boiled and reduced to produce coconut sugar, a natural sweetener with a low glycemic index. This sugar is a popular alternative to cane sugar, particularly in traditional Asian cuisine and among health-conscious consumers.

j. Coconut vinegar: The sap from the inflorescence can also be fermented to produce coconut vinegar, a tangy condiment with culinary and medicinal uses. Coconut vinegar is rich in nutrients and is believed to have numerous health benefits.

Quality Control and Safety:

Ensuring the quality and safety of coconut products is of utmost importance to protect consumer health and maintain the reputation of the industry. Good manufacturing practices (GMP), proper hygiene, and strict quality control measures should be implemented throughout the processing chain. Additionally, regular testing for contaminants, such as aflatoxins, pesticides, and heavy metals, is necessary to ensure the safety of the final products.

Waste Management and Sustainability:

Coconut processing generates various byproducts and waste materials, which can be utilized for additional applications or managed in an environmentally responsible manner. Examples include:

a. Coir pith: The leftover residue from coir processing can be used as a growing medium or soil conditioner in horticulture, thanks to its high water retention capacity and air porosity.

b. Shell-based products: Shells can be converted into charcoal, activated carbon, or used as a fuel source, reducing waste and providing additional income streams for coconut farmers.

c. Wastewater treatment: Wastewater generated during coconut processing, particularly in the production of coconut milk and oil, should be properly treated to minimize environmental impacts and meet regulatory requirements.

In conclusion, the harvesting and processing of coconuts are critical steps in converting this versatile fruit into a wide array of products that benefit consumers worldwide. The adoption of sustainable and environmentally responsible practices throughout the production chain can help ensure the long-term viability of the coconut industry and contribute to global food security and economic development.

Chapter 6: Culinary Uses of Coconuts

Coconuts are a staple ingredient in many traditional cuisines across the globe, particularly in tropical and coastal regions. The fruit's versatility and unique flavor profile make it a popular choice in both sweet and savory dishes. This chapter explores the various culinary uses of coconuts, highlighting some of the key ingredients derived from the fruit and providing examples of traditional and modern recipes that showcase the coconut's culinary potential.

Coconut Milk and Cream:

Coconut milk is a rich, creamy liquid extracted from grated coconut meat. It is a fundamental ingredient in many Southeast Asian curries, stews, and soups, imparting a rich, creamy texture and a subtle sweetness. Coconut cream, which is a thicker, more concentrated version of coconut milk, can be used in similar dishes or as a base for desserts and beverages.

Examples of dishes that use coconut milk or cream include Thai green curry, Indonesian rendang, Filipino ginataang, and Caribbean rice and peas.

Coconut Oil:

Coconut oil is a versatile cooking fat with a high smoke point, making it suitable for frying, sautéing, and baking. Its unique flavor adds a subtle coconut aroma to dishes, and it is a popular choice for vegan and paleo diets as a substitute for other fats.

Examples of dishes that use coconut oil include Sri Lankan pol sambol, Indian coconut chutney, and vegan chocolate chip cookies.

Coconut Water:

Coconut water is the clear liquid found inside young, green coconuts. It has a sweet, slightly nutty taste and is naturally hydrating, making it a popular beverage in tropical regions. Coconut water can also be used as a cooking liquid in recipes, adding a subtle sweetness and unique flavor.

Examples of dishes that use coconut water include Brazilian moqueca, Vietnamese coconut braised pork, and tropical smoothies.

Coconut Meat:

The white, fleshy part of the coconut, known as the meat or endosperm, can be eaten fresh, dried, or toasted. It is a popular ingredient in desserts, snacks, and salads, adding a chewy texture and a mildly sweet, nutty flavor.

Examples of dishes that use coconut meat include Indian coconut burfi, Thai coconut sticky rice with mango, and tropical fruit salads.

Coconut Flour:

Coconut flour is a gluten-free alternative to wheat flour, made from the residual coconut meal left after oil extraction. It has a mild coconut flavor and can be used in various baked goods and recipes, although it requires adjustments to the liquid and binding ingredients due to its high absorbency.

Examples of dishes that use coconut flour include coconut flour pancakes, coconut flour banana bread, and coconut flour cookies.

Coconut Sugar:

Coconut sugar, derived from the sap of the coconut palm's inflorescence, is a natural sweetener with a low glycemic index. It has a caramel-like flavor and can be used as a substitute for cane sugar in various recipes.

Examples of dishes that use coconut sugar include Indonesian gula melaka, coconut sugar caramel sauce, and coconut sugar-sweetened beverages.

In conclusion, coconuts offer a wide range of culinary possibilities, from rich, creamy curries to refreshing beverages and delectable desserts. The fruit's versatility, unique flavor, and nutritional benefits make it a valued ingredient in traditional cuisines and modern culinary innovations alike. As global interest in coconuts continues to grow, we can expect to see even more creative uses for this remarkable tropical fruit in kitchens around the world.

Chapter 7: Health Benefits and Medicinal Uses of Coconuts

Coconuts have been utilized for their health benefits and medicinal properties for centuries, particularly in traditional medicine systems across the globe. Recent scientific research has begun to validate many of these traditional uses, revealing the potential of coconuts to support overall health and wellbeing. This chapter explores the health benefits and medicinal uses of coconuts, focusing on the various components of the fruit and their effects on human health.

Nutritional Benefits:

Coconuts are rich in nutrients, providing an array of essential vitamins, minerals, and dietary fiber. The fruit is a good source of manganese, potassium, magnesium, and copper, as well as B vitamins and vitamin C. The high fiber content of coconuts can promote digestive health and support healthy weight management.

Fats and Heart Health:

While coconuts are high in saturated fat, the majority of this fat comes in the form of medium-chain triglycerides (MCTs), particularly lauric acid. MCTs are metabolized differently than long-chain fatty acids, providing a quick source of energy and potentially promoting weight loss. Some studies suggest that lauric acid may help increase HDL („good") cholesterol levels and improve overall cholesterol profiles, which could contribute to better heart health.

Immune Support:

Coconut oil contains antimicrobial, antifungal, and antiviral properties, primarily due to its high content of lauric acid and caprylic acid. These fatty acids may help support the immune system by combating harmful microorganisms and preventing infections. Traditional use of coconut oil includes topical application for skin infections and consumption for gastrointestinal issues caused by bacteria or parasites.

Skin and Hair Health:

Coconut oil is a popular ingredient in natural skin and hair care products, thanks to its moisturizing, antioxidant, and anti-inflammatory properties. Applying coconut oil topically can help soothe dry or irritated skin, protect against sun damage, and promote wound healing. As a hair treatment, coconut oil can help reduce protein loss, minimize damage, and improve overall hair health.

Brain Health:

The MCTs in coconut oil can be converted into ketones, which serve as an alternative fuel source for the brain. Some studies suggest that ketones may have neuroprotective effects and could help improve cognitive function in individuals with Alzheimer's disease or other neurodegenerative conditions.

Blood Sugar Control:

Coconut products, such as coconut flour and coconut sugar, have a low glycemic index, meaning they cause a slower and smaller rise in blood sugar levels compared to other carbohydrate sources. Incorporating low-glycemic foods into the diet may help manage blood sugar levels, particularly for individuals with diabetes or metabolic syndrome.

Bone and Dental Health:

The minerals found in coconuts, including calcium, phosphorus, and magnesium, play a crucial role in maintaining healthy bones and teeth. Consuming coconuts as part of a balanced diet may contribute to overall bone and dental health and help prevent osteoporosis and tooth decay.

In conclusion, coconuts offer a range of health benefits and medicinal uses, thanks to their unique nutritional profile and bioactive compounds. Incorporating coconuts and their derivatives into a balanced diet and lifestyle may support overall health and wellbeing, while their traditional medicinal uses continue to hold promise for future research and potential therapeutic applications.

Chapter 8: Industrial Applications of Coconuts

Beyond their culinary and medicinal uses, coconuts have a wide range of industrial applications. The various components of the coconut palm can be utilized in numerous industries, making it a valuable and versatile resource. This chapter explores the industrial applications of coconuts and their byproducts, highlighting their contributions to various sectors, from textiles and construction to energy and environmental sustainability.

Textiles and Fibers:

Coir, the fibrous material found between the outer husk and inner shell of the coconut, is used in the production of various textiles and fibers. Coir is strong, durable, and resistant to water and salt, making it ideal for the manufacture of ropes, mats, brushes, and upholstery padding. Additionally, coir's high lignin content makes it a suitable material for erosion control and soil stabilization applications, such as coir geotextiles and biodegradable erosion control blankets.

Construction Materials:

Coconut shells and coir can be used as raw materials in the construction industry. Coconut shells can be processed into aggregates for concrete or as a filler material for asphalt, providing a sustainable alternative to traditional aggregates. Coir, on the other hand, can be used as a component in the production of eco-friendly building materials, such as coir-based composites and insulation panels.

Energy and Biofuel:

Coconut shells and husks can be utilized as a renewable source of energy in the form of biomass. The shells can be processed into charcoal or activated carbon, which can be used as a fuel source or for various industrial applications, such as water and air purification. Additionally, the oil extracted from coconut meat can be converted into biodiesel, a renewable and environmentally friendly alternative to fossil fuels.

Biodegradable Products:

Coconuts and their byproducts can be used as raw materials for the production of biodegradable and eco-friendly products. For example, coconut shells can be turned into biodegradable packaging materials, cutlery, and dishes, offering a sustainable alternative to single-use plastics. Coir can also be used to create biodegradable pots for plants and seedlings, reducing the need for plastic containers in horticulture and landscaping.

Water Treatment:

Activated carbon derived from coconut shells is widely used in water treatment applications, thanks to its high adsorption capacity and effectiveness in removing impurities. Coconut shell-based activated carbon can be used to filter out contaminants, such as heavy metals, pesticides, and volatile organic compounds, improving the quality and safety of drinking water.

Waste Management and Sustainability:

Coconut processing generates various byproducts and waste materials, which can be utilized for additional applications or managed in an environmentally responsible manner. Examples include the use of coir pith as a growing medium or soil conditioner in horticulture and the conversion of shells into charcoal or activated carbon, reducing waste and providing additional income streams for coconut farmers.

In conclusion, coconuts and their byproducts offer a range of industrial applications that contribute to the development of sustainable and environmentally friendly solutions across various sectors. The versatility and eco-friendly nature of coconuts make them a valuable resource, helping to address global challenges, such as climate change, resource depletion, and waste management.

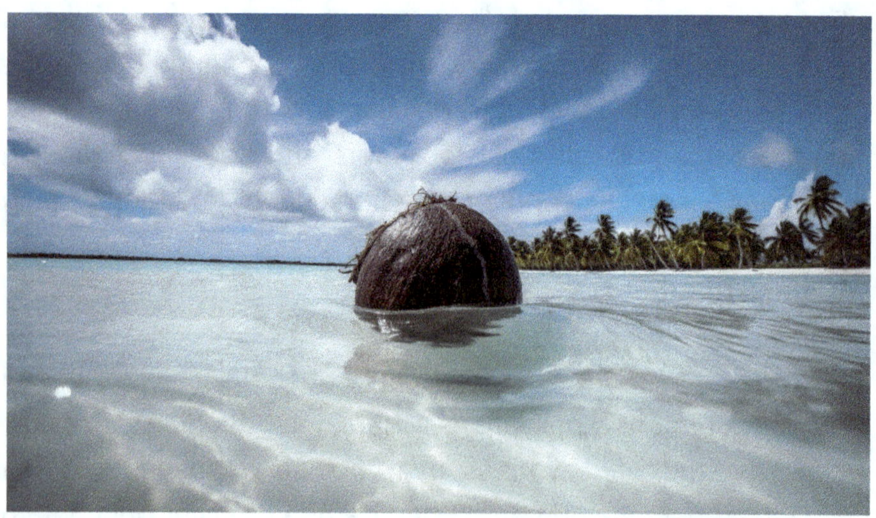

Chapter 9: Coconut-Based Beauty and Personal Care Products

The unique properties of coconuts and their derivatives make them ideal ingredients for a wide range of beauty and personal care products. Rich in nutrients, antioxidants, and fatty acids, coconut-based products can provide various benefits for skin, hair, and overall health. This chapter explores the use of coconuts in beauty and personal care products, highlighting their potential benefits and popular applications.

Coconut Oil:

Coconut oil has become a popular ingredient in natural beauty products due to its moisturizing, antioxidant, and anti-inflammatory properties. Common uses of coconut oil in personal care products include:

a. Skin care: Coconut oil can be used as a moisturizer, makeup remover, or body oil, helping to nourish and soothe dry or irritated skin. Its antimicrobial properties can also aid in the treatment of minor skin infections and acne.

b. Hair care: Coconut oil can be used as a pre-shampoo treatment, hair mask, or leave-in conditioner to help repair damaged hair, reduce protein loss, and improve overall hair health.

c. Oral care: Coconut oil can be used for oil pulling, an ancient Ayurvedic practice that involves swishing oil in the mouth to remove bacteria, promote oral hygiene, and whiten teeth.

Coconut Water:

Coconut water, the clear liquid found inside young, green coconuts, is rich in electrolytes, vitamins, and minerals. It is used in various beauty products for its hydrating and revitalizing properties, such as:

a. Facial mists and toners: Coconut water can be used as a base for facial mists and toners, providing hydration and a refreshing feel for the skin.

b. Hair care products: Coconut water can be incorporated into shampoos, conditioners, and hair treatments for added hydration and nourishment.

Coconut Milk and Cream:

The rich, creamy texture of coconut milk and cream makes them ideal ingredients for moisturizing and nourishing personal care products, such as:

a. Body lotions and creams: Coconut milk and cream can be used as a base for body lotions and creams, providing deep hydration and a luxurious feel for the skin.

b. Hair masks and treatments: Coconut milk and cream can be used in hair masks and deep conditioning treatments to restore moisture, shine, and softness to dry or damaged hair.

Coconut-Derived Surfactants:

Surfactants derived from coconuts, such as sodium coco-sulfate and cocamidopropyl betaine, are commonly used in natural and eco-friendly personal care products. These coconut-derived surfactants are used as alternatives to harsher synthetic surfactants in products like shampoos, body washes, and facial cleansers.

Coconut Shell Activated Charcoal:

Activated charcoal derived from coconut shells has become a popular ingredient in beauty products for its detoxifying and purifying properties. Common applications of coconut shell activated charcoal include:

a. Face masks and cleansers: Activated charcoal can be used in face masks and cleansers to help draw out impurities, unclog pores, and detoxify the skin.

b. Oral care products: Activated charcoal can be used in toothpaste and tooth powders to help remove surface stains, whiten teeth, and promote overall oral hygiene.

In conclusion, coconuts and their byproducts offer a wealth of benefits for beauty and personal care applications. From nourishing skin and hair to promoting oral hygiene and detoxification, coconut-based products provide natural, effective, and eco-friendly alternatives to conventional personal care items. As the demand for sustainable and clean beauty products continues to grow, the use of coconuts in this industry is likely to expand and innovate further.

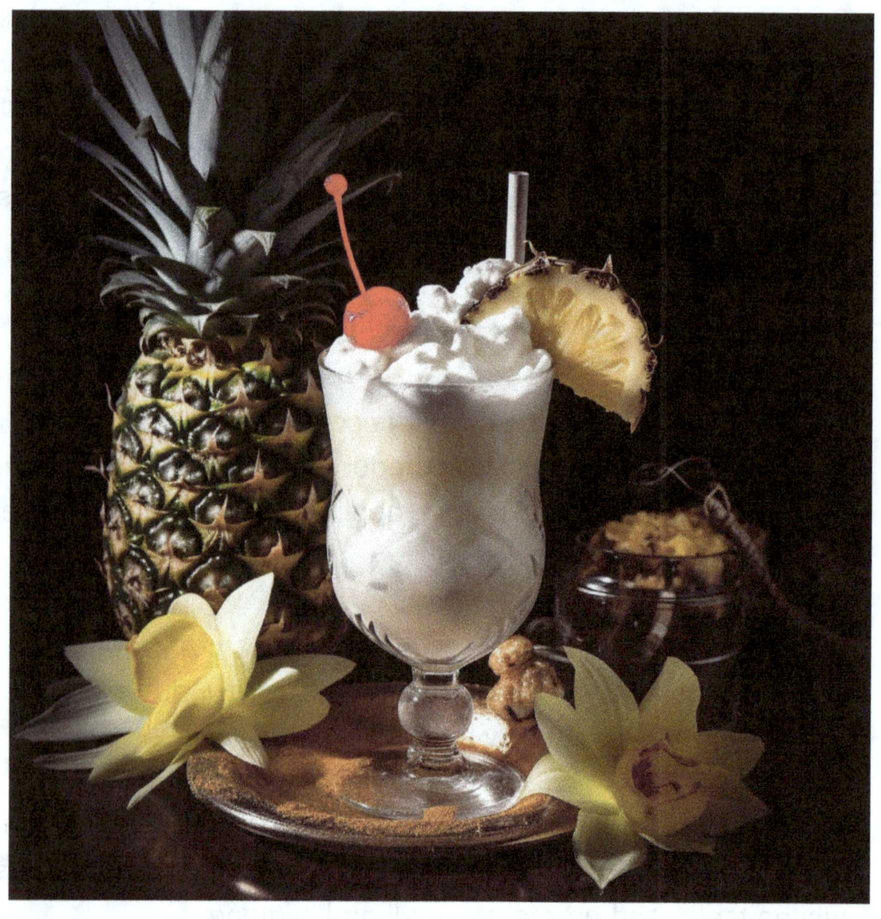

Piña Colada, a base de zumo de piña, ron blanco y leche de coco

Chapter 10: Environmental Impact and Sustainability of Coconut Production

As the global demand for coconuts and their byproducts continues to grow, it becomes increasingly important to consider the environmental impact and sustainability of coconut production. This chapter discusses the environmental implications of coconut cultivation, the potential challenges faced by the industry, and the ways in which sustainable practices can be implemented to minimize negative effects and promote responsible growth.

Positive Environmental Impacts:

Coconut palms have several characteristics that contribute to their positive environmental impact. Some of these include:

a. Carbon sequestration: Coconut palms can act as carbon sinks, absorbing carbon dioxide from the atmosphere and converting it into biomass, which helps mitigate climate change.

b. Erosion control: The extensive root systems of coconut palms help stabilize soil, prevent erosion, and protect coastal areas from storm surges and rising sea levels.

c. Biodiversity: Coconut plantations can support a diverse range of plant and animal species, contributing to ecosystem health and resilience.

d. Renewable resource: Coconuts are a renewable resource, with each palm producing fruit for up to 60 years. Furthermore, nearly every part of the coconut palm can be utilized, reducing waste and promoting resource efficiency.

Potential Environmental Challenges:

Despite these positive attributes, there are potential environmental challenges associated with coconut production, such as:

a. Deforestation: The expansion of coconut plantations can lead to deforestation and habitat loss if not managed responsibly.

b. Pesticide and fertilizer use: The use of chemical pesticides and fertilizers in coconut cultivation can have negative impacts on soil, water, and ecosystems, threatening biodiversity and human health.

c. Monoculture: The practice of growing a single crop species over large areas can reduce biodiversity, leading to soil degradation, nutrient depletion, and increased vulnerability to pests and diseases.

Promoting Sustainability in Coconut Production:

To mitigate potential environmental challenges and ensure the sustainability of coconut production, several strategies can be implemented:

a. Agroforestry and intercropping: Integrating coconut palms with other crops or tree species can improve biodiversity, soil health, and pest management, while providing additional income streams for farmers.

b. Organic and regenerative farming practices: Adopting organic and regenerative practices, such as minimizing chemical inputs, conserving water, and enhancing soil fertility, can reduce the environmental impact of coconut cultivation and promote long-term productivity.

c. Fair trade and ethical sourcing: Supporting fair trade and ethical sourcing initiatives can help ensure that coconut farmers receive fair compensation for their products, encouraging the adoption of sustainable farming practices and improving the livelihoods of farming communities.

d. Waste management and resource efficiency: Utilizing waste products from coconut processing, such as shells and husks, for energy production or other industrial applications can reduce waste and promote resource efficiency.

e. Reforestation and habitat conservation: Ensuring that the expansion of coconut plantations is conducted responsibly, with minimal impact on forests and habitats, is crucial for protecting biodiversity and ecosystem services.

In conclusion, the environmental impact and sustainability of coconut production are complex issues that require a balanced approach. By implementing sustainable practices, promoting responsible sourcing, and supporting the livelihoods of coconut farming communities, the coconut industry can continue to grow while minimizing negative environmental impacts and contributing to global sustainability goals.

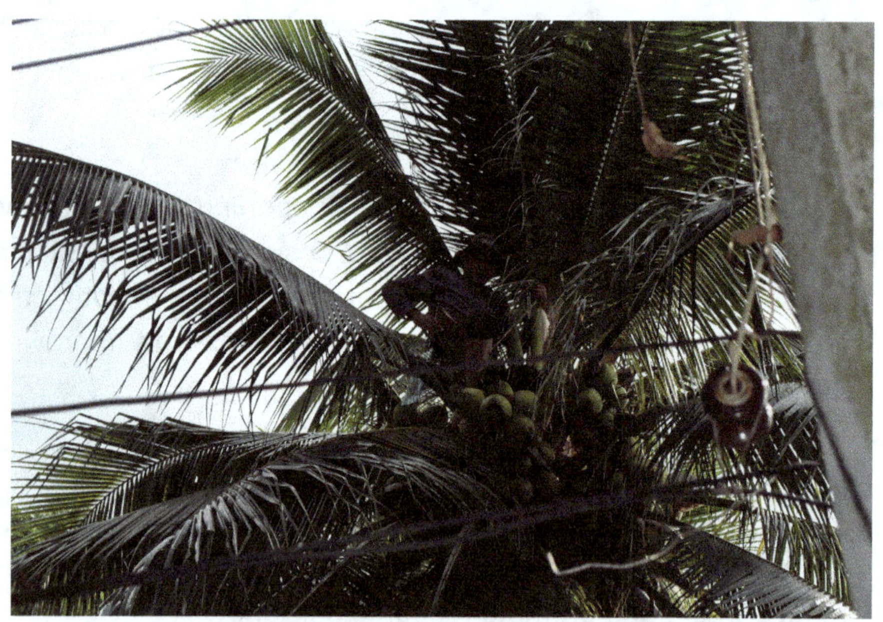

Coconut picker at work in about 15 meters height, here in Thailand

Chapter 11: The Role of Coconuts in Culture and Folklore

Throughout history, coconuts have played a significant role in the culture and folklore of various societies across the globe. Revered for their versatility, coconuts have been used as symbols of fertility, prosperity, and life. This chapter explores the cultural significance and rich folklore surrounding coconuts, shedding light on their influence in art, religion, and storytelling.

Coconuts in Mythology and Religion:

Coconuts have been associated with numerous myths and religious beliefs across different cultures. For example:

a. Hinduism: In Hindu rituals, coconuts are often used as offerings to deities, symbolizing purity and the breaking of one's ego. The coconut is also associated with Lord Ganesha, the remover of obstacles, and is used during festivals and ceremonies as a symbol of prosperity.

b. Polynesian Culture: In Polynesian mythology, the coconut palm is considered the „Tree of Life," providing food, shelter, and tools for survival. Legends tell of the god Tane, who brought the coconut palm to earth, ensuring the well-being of the people.

c. Filipino Folklore: In Filipino folklore, the coconut palm is believed to have been created by a benevolent spirit who wanted to provide a versatile and abundant resource for humans.

Coconuts in Art and Symbolism:

The coconut has been a popular subject in art and a symbol of various cultural themes. Some examples include:

a. Traditional Art: Coconuts and coconut palms have been depicted in traditional art forms such as textiles, carvings, and paintings, often symbolizing fertility, abundance, and life.

b. Contemporary Art: In modern art, coconuts have been used as a symbol of cultural identity, nostalgia, and a connection to one's roots, particularly for artists from coconut-producing regions.

Coconuts in Folktales and Storytelling:

Folktales and stories featuring coconuts have been passed down through generations, reflecting the cultural significance and practical importance of this versatile fruit. Some examples include:

a. Indian Folktales: In Indian folktales, coconuts are often used as a symbol of wisdom, with stories teaching the value of resourcefulness and clever thinking.

b. Caribbean Folktales: In Caribbean folklore, the coconut is sometimes personified as a character in stories, often highlighting the importance of cooperation and community.

Coconuts in Festivals and Celebrations:

Coconuts play a significant role in various festivals and celebrations, often symbolizing abundance, prosperity, and new beginnings. For example:

a. Pongal (India): During the Pongal festival in South India, coconuts are offered to the sun god as a symbol of gratitude for a bountiful harvest.

b. Kwanzaa (African Diaspora): During Kwanzaa, a celebration of African heritage and culture, coconuts are used to represent the principle of „Ujamaa" or cooperative economics, emphasizing the importance of community support and shared prosperity.

In conclusion, coconuts have long held a prominent place in the culture and folklore of various societies around the world. Their versatility and practical importance have made them a powerful symbol of life, fertility, and abundance. As the global demand for coconuts continues to grow, it is essential to recognize and preserve the rich cultural heritage associated with this remarkable fruit.

Chapter 12: The Future of Coconuts: New Discoveries and Innovations

As the demand for coconuts and their byproducts continues to rise, researchers and innovators are constantly exploring new ways to utilize this versatile resource. This chapter discusses some of the emerging discoveries and innovations in the field of coconut research and development, showcasing the potential future applications of coconuts in various industries.

Biodegradable Materials:

One promising area of innovation is the development of biodegradable materials derived from coconut waste, such as husks, shells, and fibers. These materials have the potential to replace single-use plastics and synthetic materials, reducing environmental pollution and promoting a circular economy. Examples include:

a. Biodegradable packaging: Researchers are exploring the use of coconut fibers and other waste products to create eco-friendly packaging materials that can break down naturally over time.

b. Sustainable textiles: Coconut waste can be transformed into sustainable textiles, offering an alternative to synthetic fibers and reducing the environmental impact of the fashion industry.

Renewable Energy:

Coconuts can play a significant role in the transition towards renewable energy sources. Some potential applications include:

a. Biofuel production: Coconut oil can be converted into bio-diesel, offering a renewable and eco-friendly alternative to fossil fuels.

b. Biogas generation: The anaerobic digestion of coconut waste can produce biogas, a renewable source of energy that can be used for heating, cooking, and electricity generation.

Advanced Food and Beverage Applications:

In the food and beverage industry, coconuts and their byproducts are being utilized in innovative ways to cater to evolving consumer preferences and dietary needs. Examples include:

a. Plant-based dairy alternatives: Coconut milk, cream, and yogurt are becoming popular dairy alternatives for those seeking plant-based or lactose-free options.

b. Functional foods and beverages: Researchers are investigating the potential health benefits of coconut-derived ingredients, such as medium-chain triglycerides (MCTs) and lauric acid, which may be incorporated into functional foods and beverages to promote health and wellness.

Medical and Biotechnological Applications:

Coconuts and their byproducts offer potential for medical and biotechnological advancements, including:

a. Wound care: Coconut oil and its derivatives, such as monolaurin, have antimicrobial properties that may be harnessed for wound care and infection prevention.

b. Drug delivery systems: Researchers are investigating the use of coconut-derived materials, such as nanocarriers, for targeted drug delivery in medical treatments.

Genetic and Agricultural Innovations:

In order to meet the growing global demand for coconuts and ensure long-term sustainability, researchers are exploring genetic and agricultural innovations, such as:

a. Disease-resistant cultivars: Developing and promoting disease-resistant coconut varieties can help protect the global coconut supply from devastating pests and diseases.

b. Climate-resilient varieties: As climate change poses challenges to agricultural productivity, the development of climate-resilient coconut varieties will become increasingly important to ensure a sustainable supply.

In conclusion, the future of coconuts is filled with potential and exciting opportunities. As new discoveries and innovations emerge, coconuts and their byproducts will continue to contribute to a more sustainable, healthier, and eco-friendly world.

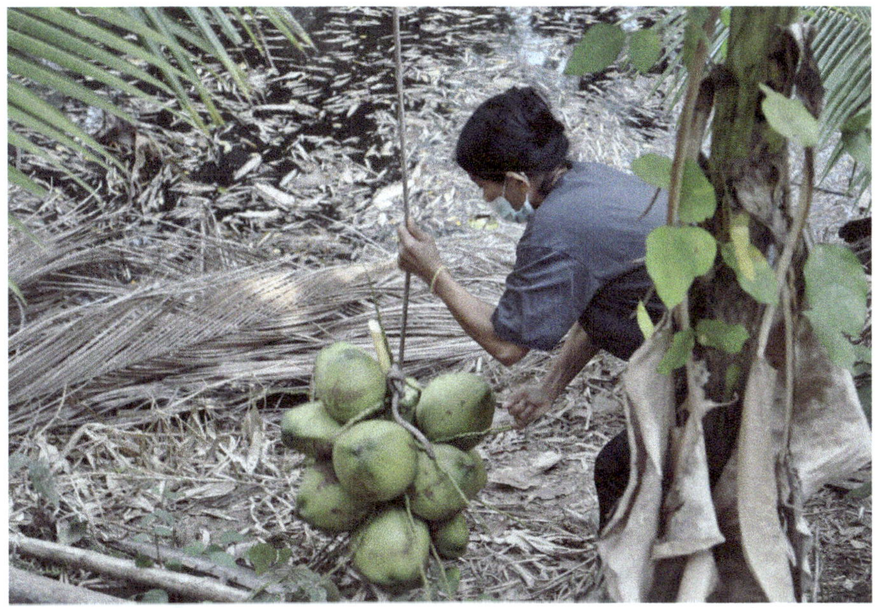

Gentle hand picking in Thailand

Chapter 13: Supporting Small Coconut Producers and Fair Trade Practices

Small coconut producers play a vital role in the global coconut industry, contributing to the livelihoods of millions of farmers and their families. However, they often face challenges such as low prices, lack of access to resources, and vulnerability to market fluctuations. This chapter explores the importance of supporting small coconut producers and promoting fair trade practices to ensure the long-term sustainability and equitable growth of the coconut industry.

Challenges Faced by Small Coconut Producers:

Small coconut producers often face several challenges, including:

a. _Price volatility:_ Fluctuations in coconut prices can have a significant impact on small producers, making it difficult for them to plan for the future and invest in their farms.

b. _Limited access to resources:_ Small producers may lack access to resources such as credit, agricultural inputs, and technical assistance, hindering their ability to adopt sustainable farming practices and improve productivity.

c. _Market access:_ Small producers may struggle to access profitable markets, leaving them vulnerable to middlemen who may offer lower prices for their products.

The Role of Fair Trade in Supporting Small Producers:

Fair trade initiatives aim to promote equitable trading relationships, ensuring that producers receive a fair price for their products and have access to the resources needed to improve their livelihoods. Some key principles of fair trade in the context of coconut production include:

a. Fair pricing: Fair trade organizations establish a minimum price for coconuts, protecting producers from price volatility and ensuring that they receive a stable income.

b. Social premiums: In addition to the minimum price, fair trade organizations often provide a social premium, which is invested in community development projects such as education, healthcare, and infrastructure.

c. Capacity building: Fair trade initiatives support small producers by providing access to training, resources, and technical assistance, enabling them to adopt sustainable farming practices and improve productivity.

d. Direct trade relationships: By establishing direct trade relationships between producers and buyers, fair trade initiatives can help small producers access profitable markets and negotiate better prices for their products.

Empowering Small Producers through Cooperatives:

Forming cooperatives can be an effective way for small coconut producers to pool resources, access markets, and negotiate better prices for their products. Some benefits of cooperatives include:

a. Collective bargaining power: Cooperatives can help small producers negotiate better prices and terms with buyers, reducing their vulnerability to market fluctuations.

b. Shared resources and knowledge: Cooperatives can facilitate the sharing of resources and knowledge among members, enabling small producers to adopt sustainable farming practices and improve productivity.

c. Access to credit and financing: By pooling resources, cooperatives can help small producers access credit and financing, which can be used to invest in farm improvements, equipment, and infrastructure.

In conclusion, supporting small coconut producers and promoting fair trade practices are crucial for ensuring the long-term sustainability and equitable growth of the coconut industry. By empowering small producers through fair trade initiatives and cooperatives, we can create a more resilient and inclusive coconut industry that benefits both producers and consumers.

Chapter 14: Delicious Coconut Recipes to Try at Home

Coconuts are a versatile and delicious ingredient that can be incorporated into a wide variety of dishes. In this chapter, we will explore some delightful coconut recipes that showcase the diverse culinary applications of this remarkable fruit. From sweet treats to savory dishes, these recipes are sure to inspire you to get creative in the kitchen.

Coconut Curry:

A rich and flavorful coconut curry is a perfect way to showcase the creaminess and subtle sweetness of coconut milk. Combine coconut milk with your choice of vegetables, protein (such as chicken, tofu, or shrimp), and a blend of aromatic spices, such as curry powder, cumin, coriander, and turmeric. Serve over steamed rice or with warm naan bread for a satisfying and comforting meal.

Coconut Rice:

Coconut rice is a delicious side dish that pairs well with a variety of entrees. To prepare, simply cook jasmine or basmati rice with coconut milk, water, and a pinch of salt. For added flavor, you can also include aromatics such as lemongrass, ginger, or pandan leaves.

Coconut Shrimp:

For a tropical twist on a classic appetizer, try coconut shrimp. Coat peeled and deveined shrimp in a mixture of flour, beaten egg, and shredded coconut, then fry until golden brown. Serve with a tangy dipping sauce, such as sweet chili sauce or mango salsa, for a crowd-pleasing dish.

Coconut Macaroons:

These sweet and chewy treats are a coconut lover's dream. Combine shredded coconut, sweetened condensed milk, and vanilla extract, then shape into small mounds and bake until lightly golden. For an extra touch of decadence, dip the cooled macaroons in melted chocolate.

Coconut Smoothie:

A coconut smoothie is a refreshing and nourishing beverage that's perfect for a quick breakfast or snack. Blend coconut milk, fresh or frozen fruit (such as pineapple, mango, or banana), and a handful of ice until smooth. For added nutrition, you can also include a scoop of protein powder, a spoonful of chia seeds, or a handful of spinach.

Coconut Soup (Tom Kha Gai):

This Thai-inspired coconut soup is a deliciously fragrant and comforting dish. Simmer coconut milk with chicken broth, lemongrass, galangal, and kaffir lime leaves, then add sliced chicken, mushrooms, and fish sauce for a savory, tangy flavor. Finish with a squeeze of fresh lime juice and a handful of chopped cilantro for a burst of brightness.

Coconut Chutney:

Coconut chutney is a popular accompaniment to South Indian dishes such as dosas and idlis. To prepare, grind grated coconut, green chilies, ginger, and roasted chana dal (split chickpeas) in a blender or food processor, then season with salt, tamarind paste, and a splash of water. For a traditional tadka (tempering), heat oil in a small pan, then add mustard seeds, curry leaves, and dried red chilies, and pour over the chutney.

In conclusion, coconuts offer a wealth of culinary possibilities that can be enjoyed in sweet and savory dishes alike. These recipes are just a starting point for your own culinary adventures with this versatile and delicious fruit.

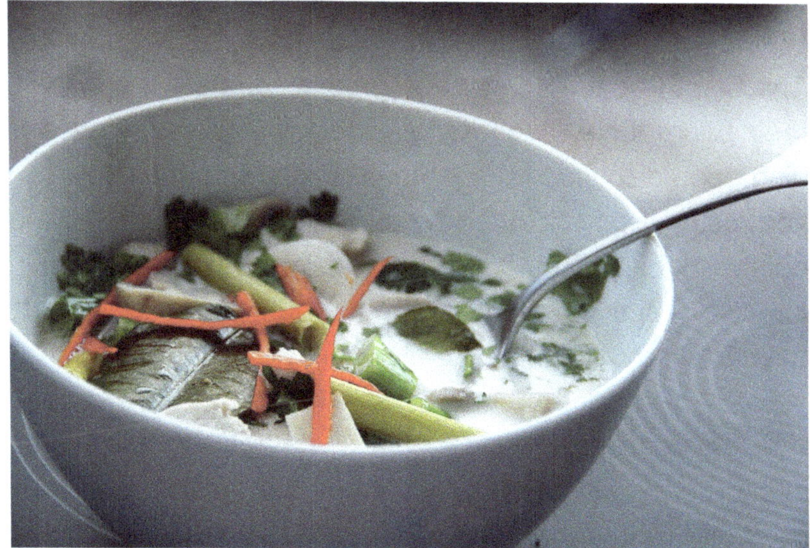

„Tom Kha Gai"

Chapter 15: Conclusion: Embracing the Versatility of Coconuts

Throughout this book, we have explored the remarkable world of coconuts, delving into their history, cultivation, and numerous applications in various industries. From their origins in the Indo-Pacific region to their global spread and integration into diverse cultures, coconuts have proven to be an incredibly versatile and valuable resource.

As we have seen, coconuts play a crucial role in the livelihoods of millions of people, particularly small producers who depend on this crop for their income and sustenance. Supporting these producers through fair trade practices and cooperatives is essential for ensuring the long-term sustainability and equitable growth of the coconut industry.

The health benefits and nutritional properties of coconuts and their byproducts, such as coconut oil, milk, and water, have also been discussed. These products are increasingly recognized for their potential to promote wellness and contribute to a balanced diet. Furthermore, coconuts have found their way into the realm of beauty and personal care products, offering natural alternatives to synthetic ingredients.

The environmental impact and sustainability of coconut production have also been a key focus, as the industry continues to evolve and adopt more eco-friendly practices. By utilizing coconut waste and developing innovative applications, we can create a more circular and sustainable economy.

Innovations in the field of coconuts have led to exciting new discoveries and applications, such as biodegradable materials, renewable energy sources, and advanced food and beverage products. As research and development continue, we can expect to see even more creative and groundbreaking uses for this incredible resource.

Finally, we have explored the culinary versatility of coconuts, sharing delicious recipes that showcase the diverse flavors and textures that coconuts can bring to our tables. These recipes are just a small sample of the countless ways in which coconuts can be incorporated into our meals, offering a taste of the tropics in every bite.

In conclusion, the world of coconuts is vast and diverse, offering endless possibilities for innovation, sustainability, and enjoyment. By embracing the versatility of coconuts and supporting sustainable practices, we can contribute to a more resilient and inclusive global coconut industry that benefits both producers and consumers alike. As we continue to discover new applications and appreciate the many gifts that coconuts have to offer, we can truly celebrate the remarkable journey of this extraordinary fruit.

Disclaimer

This book is intended for informational and educational purposes only and is not intended as a substitute for professional advice. While the author has made every effort to ensure the accuracy and completeness of the information contained within this book, no guarantee or warranty, expressed or implied, is made as to its accuracy or completeness. The author and publisher assume no responsibility for any errors, omissions, or for any consequences resulting from the use of the information provided.

The information contained within this book should not be used for diagnosing or treating a health problem or disease, nor should it be used as a substitute for professional medical advice, diagnosis, or treatment. Always consult a qualified healthcare professional before making any changes to your diet, exercise, or lifestyle, or before taking any supplements, medications, or making any decisions about your health.

The recipes and culinary suggestions in this book are provided for general informational purposes only and should be used at the reader's discretion. The author and publisher are not responsible for any adverse reactions, allergies, or health issues that may result from the consumption of the ingredients or dishes mentioned in this book.

The views and opinions expressed in this book are those of the author and do not necessarily reflect the official policy or position of any other agency, organization, employer, or company. Any references to specific products, brands, or companies are for illustrative purposes only and do not constitute an endorsement or recommendation.

The author and publisher do not assume any liability or responsibility for any loss, damage, or injury, including death, that may result from the use or misuse of the information contained in this book. The reader assumes full responsibility for their actions and choices related to the contents of this book.

Other books by the author

Neanderthals: Unraveling the Secrets of Our Ancient Relatives

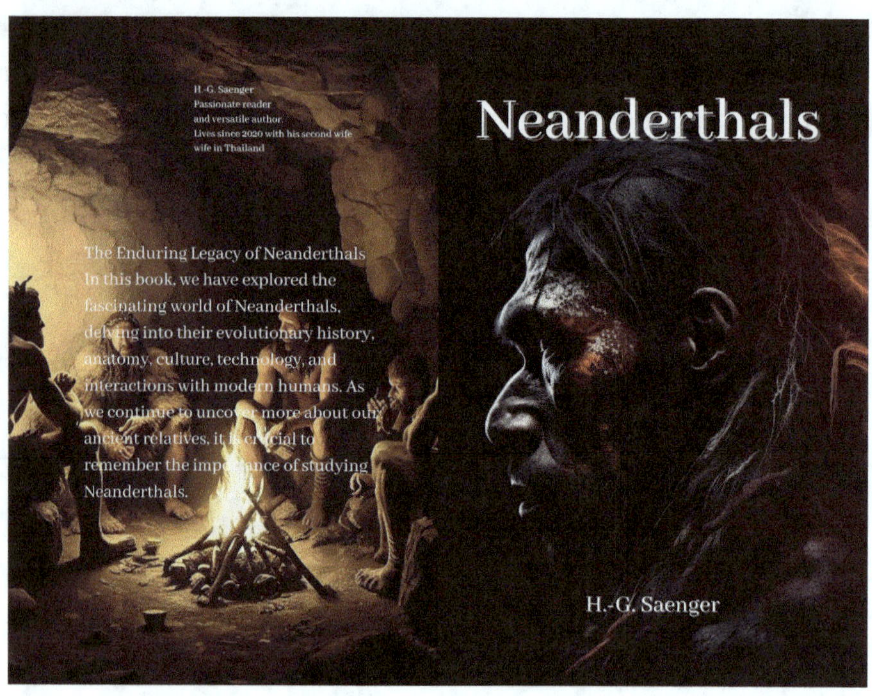

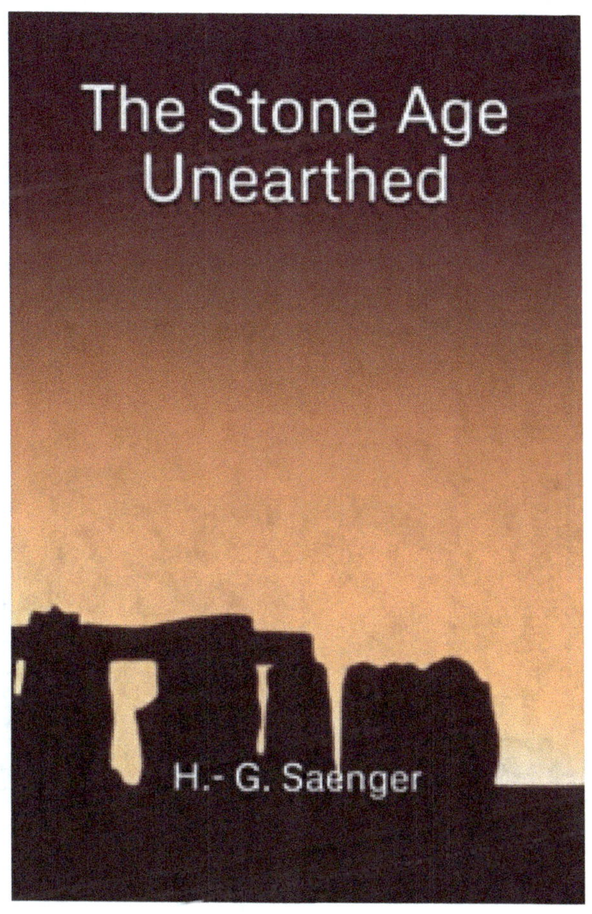
The Stone Age
Unearthed
H.- G. Saenger

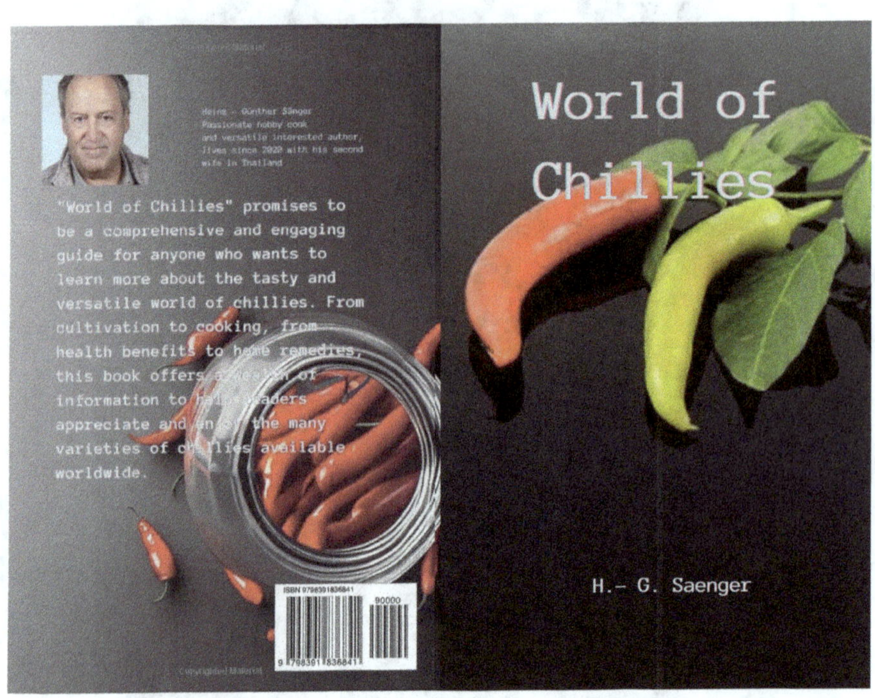
World of Chillies

H. – G. Saenger

Heinz – Günther Sänger
Passionate hobby cook
and versatile interested author,
lives since 2020 with his second
wife in Thailand

"World of Chillies" promises to
be a comprehensive and engaging
guide for anyone who wants to
learn more about the tasty and
versatile world of chillies. From
cultivation to cooking, from
health benefits to home remedies,
this book offers a wealth of
information to help readers
appreciate and enjoy the many
varieties of chillies available
worldwide.

ISBN 9798391836841

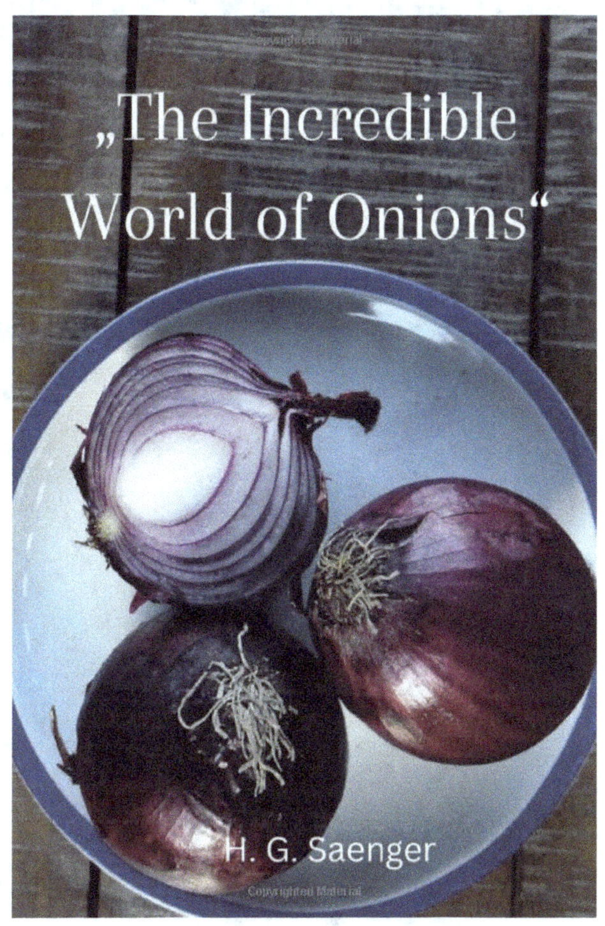

„The Incredible
World of Onions"
H. G. Saenger

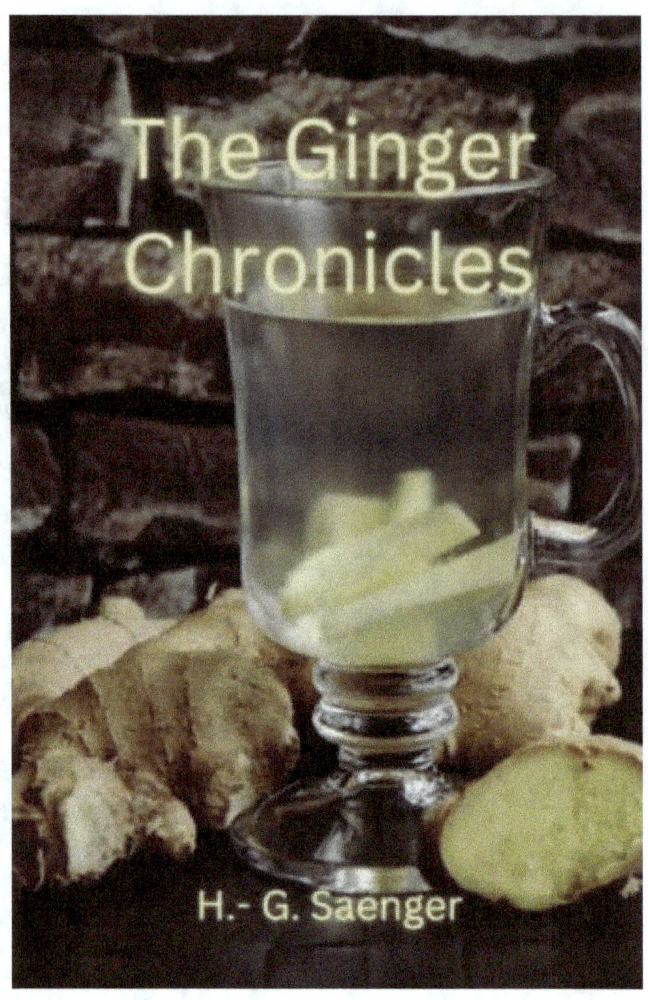
The Ginger
Chronicles
H.- G. Saenger

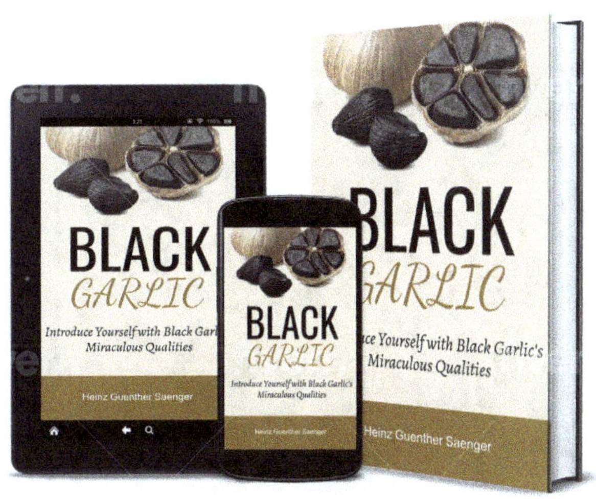
BLACK
GARLIC
Introduce Yourself with Black Garlic's
Miraculous Qualities
Heinz Guenther Saenger

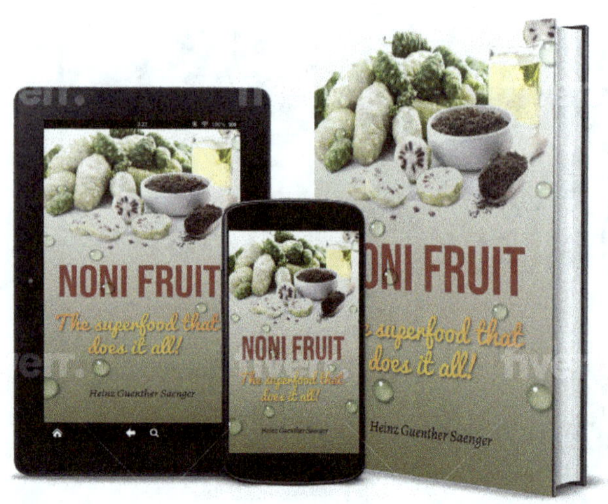

NONI FRUIT
The superfood that does it all!
Heinz Guenther Saenger
NONI FRUIT
The superfood that does it all!
Heinz Guenther Saenger
NONI FRUIT
The superfood that does it all!
Heinz Guenther Saenger

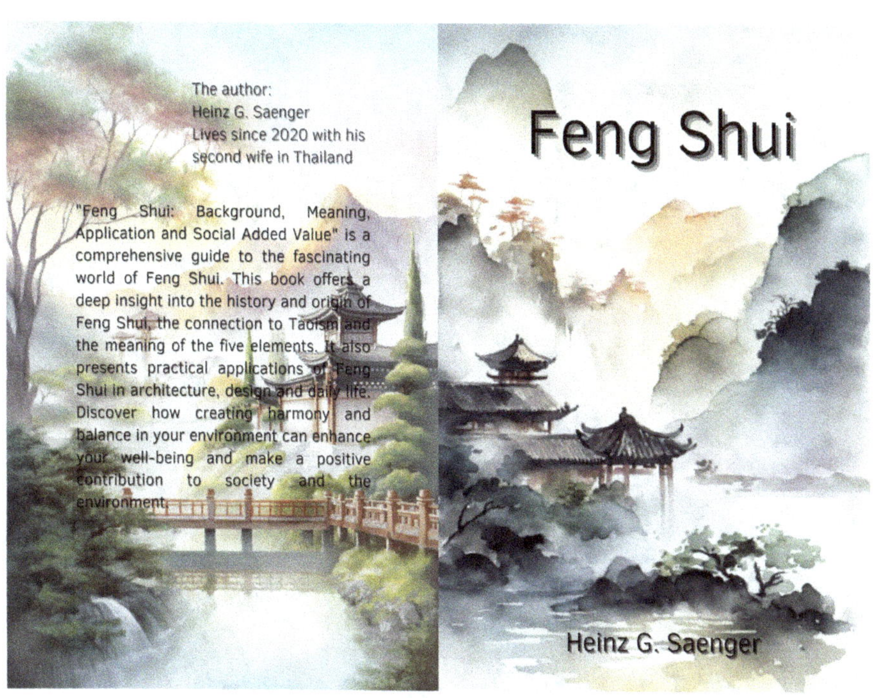
The author:
Heinz G. Saenger
Lives since 2020 with his
second wife in Thailand

"Feng Shui: Background, Meaning,
Application and Social Added Value" is a
comprehensive guide to the fascinating
world of Feng Shui. This book offers a
deep insight into the history and origin of
Feng Shui, the connection to Taoism and
the meaning of the five elements. It also
presents practical applications of Feng
Shui in architecture, design and daily life.
Discover how creating harmony and
balance in your environment can enhance
your well-being and make a positive
contribution to society and the
environment.

Feng Shui

Heinz G. Saenger

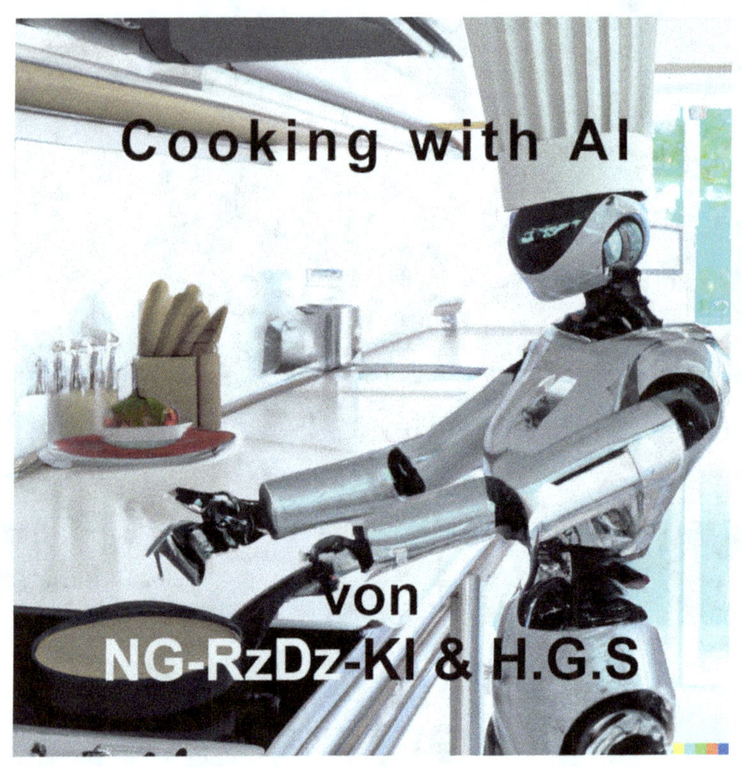
Cooking with AI
von
NG-RzDz-KI & H.G.S

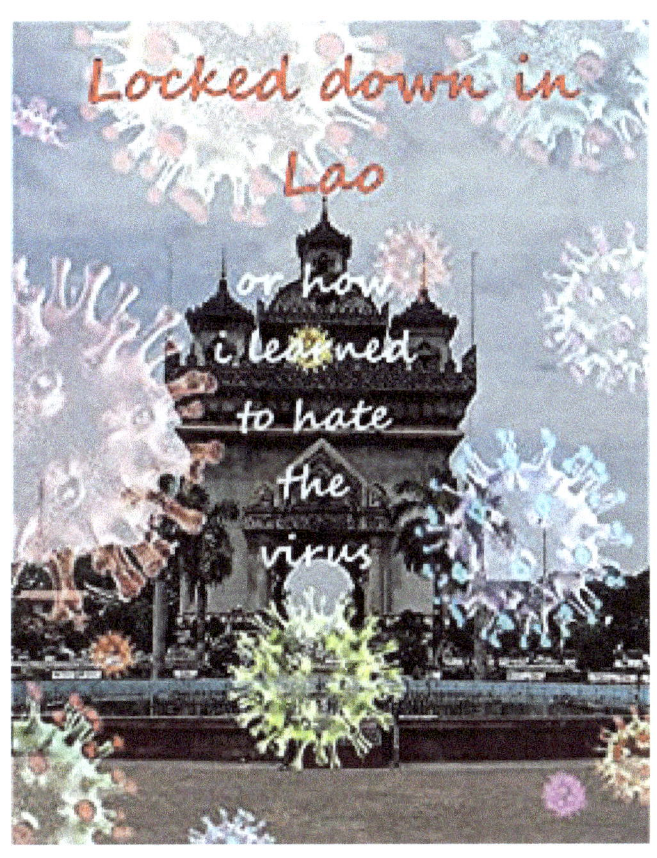

Locked down in
Lao
or how
i learned
to hate
the
virus

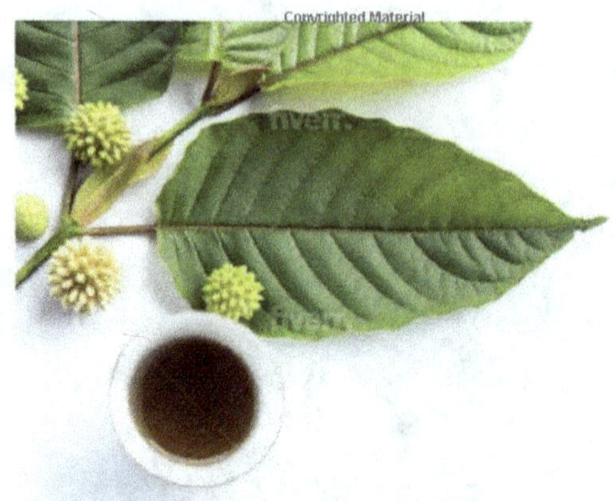

KRATOM FOR NEWBIES

All You Need To Know About Kratom Usage

By Heinz Guenther Saenger

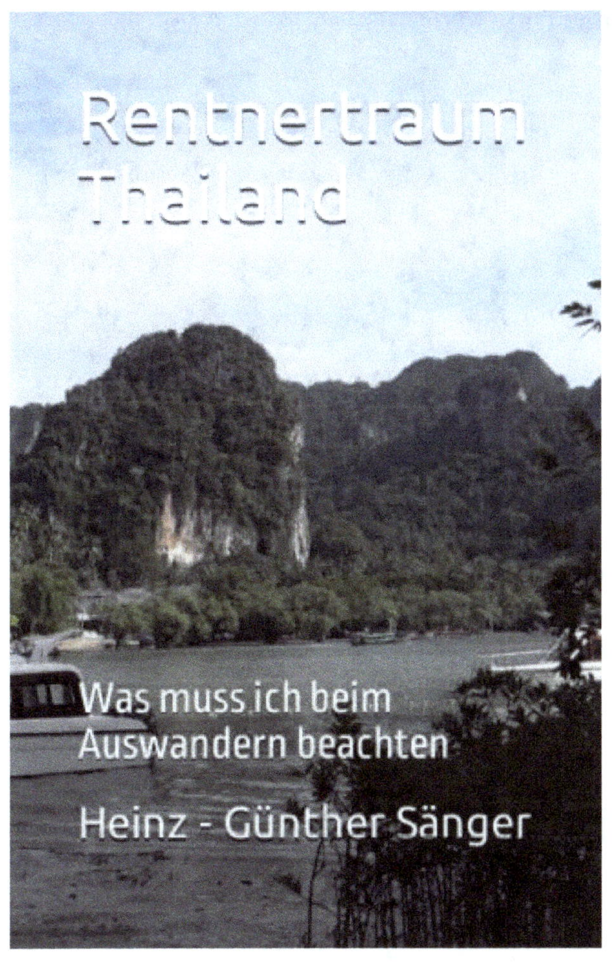
Rentnertraum
Thailand
Was muss ich beim
Auswandern beachten
Heinz - Günther Sänger

Turmeric: The Golden Treasure of Asia

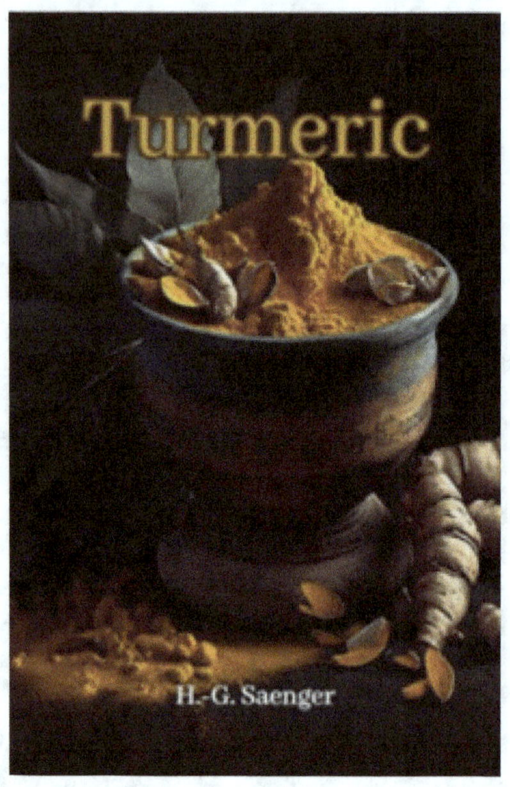